Dialysis Essential & Its System Elements

Dialysis Equipments

WALKER GUERRIER

Dialysis Essential & Its System Elements
Dialysis Equipments
All Rights Reserved.
Copyright © 2020 Walker Guerrier
v1.0

The opinions expressed in this manuscript are solely the opinions of the author and do not represent the opinions or thoughts of the publisher. The author has represented and warranted full ownership and/or legal right to publish all the materials in this book.

This book may not be reproduced, transmitted, or stored in whole or in part by any means, including graphic, electronic, or mechanical without the express written consent of the publisher except in the case of brief quotations embodied in critical articles and reviews.

Outskirts Press, Inc.
http://www.outskirtspress.com

ISBN: 978-1-9772-2510-8

Cover Photo © 2020 Walker Guerrier. All rights reserved - used with permission.

Outskirts Press and the "OP" logo are trademarks belonging to Outskirts Press, Inc.

PRINTED IN THE UNITED STATES OF AMERICA

If interested in ordering any of our products please contact us at:
www.wufotechnologies.com OR
walkergue@gmail.com

Covid-19 is also known as the coronavirus. In January 2020 as everyone had just finished celebrating the New Year, we received the news of this virus making a touchdown in our homeland, the United States. For many this was like a horror movie; we also learned that this virus is more dangerous than the common flu, and there is no known cure for it.

This virus started in some part of the world and spread almost all over the world, and we know our lives may never be the same. Just within a few months this virus spread to more than 1.3 million people in the world, killing more than ,100.000. Right here in the United States there are more than 462,000 cases and at least 100,000 deaths in the U.S. For sure it was the great effort and guidance of our mayor and governor that prevented our situation from becoming total chaos. Maybe millions of Americans would have died. It was their reinforcement of stay-at-home guidelines that saved many lives. Our world may never get to normal if we don't undo what this virus has done. For this we will need a vaccine to protect the world and its population.

This has become a race against time.

From this moment on our best course to fight this virus is to makes strategic moves which are offensive and defensive. The defensive move is to stay at home, and the offensive is to start looking at anti-viral medication we are currently using, including blood plasma of people who have immunity. For those who are not sure how dangerous this virus is, here are some of the facts. This virus not only damages the lungs; in addition it may also cause other internal damage such as heart damage, inflammation, neurological malfunction, blood clots, and intestinal damage to the liver and other organs.

What makes this virus so dangerous?

Patients may arrive at the emergency room with respiratory complications after being treated and seem to be doing well, but a few hours later they start developing cardiac issues, which are not related to respiration. At this point our brain does what it does best, causing our immune to shift its defense to hyperdrive. When this happens, our body starts to release a substance called cytokine. At this point the patient's immune system is using and doing everything it can to save the person's life. If that does not help, the other procedure to save the person is intensive—ventilation.

What are some of the symptoms of Covid-19?

- Loss of sense of smell
- Respiratory issues
- Fever
- Confusion
- Low blood oxygen level
- Loss of consciousness

Hygiene advice: clean hands frequently

YOUR DIET

Your diet plays a major role and helps reverse damage to your organs such as lungs, liver, and kidneys.

Most people don't think that their diet plays a role in helping to reverse their organ damage, and eating the wrong food could cause damage to the affected organs. Choosing the right food to eat can help your organs' health if you have had Covid-19 or have kidney damage. Consuming good food can improve your kidney function.

What are some effective renal diets that can help?

Eating food that your digestive system and kidneys have a hard time digesting would cause more damage to your kidneys, such as food that contains too much potassium, phosphorus, or sodium. These can do serious damage to your kidneys; in addition a bad diet can cause other health problems for you such as high blood pressure. Minimize your intake of soda and coffee, as these can give you more complications.

I strongly believe you should discuss this with your health care provider to learn more about the diet choices that are best for you in regard to specific kidney problems and treatment plans.

Food that Heals the Kidneys:

- Strawberry
- Kiwi
- Blueberry

These have free radicals that can reverse the kidney's cell damage.

THE SYSTEM ELEMENTS

PATENT A
511893709

Medical Bed — brief description of the drawings

Fig. 1 is a perspective view of the invention in use.

Fig. 2 is a close-up view of the invention.

Fig. 3 is a front view of the invention.

Fig. 4 is a perspective view of the invention illustrating the hinge pin being removed.

Fig. 5 is a perspective view of the bed illustrating the side panel and side panel base platform being removed.

Fig. 6 is a perspective view of the invention shown in use, illustrating the active platform being moved; side panel and side panel base platform removed for clarity.

Fig. 7 is a side view of the invention illustrating the active platform being moved; side panel l and side panel base platform removed for clarity.

Fig. 8 is a perspective view of the needle adjuster.

Fig. 9 is a close-up view of the needle adjuster.

Fig. 10 is a top view of the needle adjuster.

Fig. 11 is a side view of the needle adjuster.

Fig. 12 is a front view of the needle adjuster.

Fig. 13 is a rear view of the needle adjuster.

Fig. 14 is a section view of the needle adjuster taken 14-14 in Fig 8.

Fig. 15 is a perspective view of the armrest shown in use.

Fig. 16 is a perspective view of the armrest.

Fig. 17 is a perspective view of the pants illustrating the zipper closed.

Fig. 18 is a perspective view of the pants illustrating the zipper opened, shown in use and shirt in use.

Fig. 19 is a perspective view of the cleaning system, the perspective tray, and the tray supports shown in use.

Fig. 20 is a close-up view of the cleaning system, the prescription tray, and the tray supports.

Fig. 21 is a side view of the cleaning system, the prescription tray, and the tray supports shown in use.

Fig. 22 is a close-up view of the prescription tray.

DETAILED DESCRIPTION OF THE INVENTION: The following detailed description is of the best currently contemplated modes of carrying out exemplary embodiments of the invention. The description is not to be taken in a limiting sense, but is made merely for the purpose of illustrating the general principles of the invention. The invention is a sliding bed for medical use for all patients.

The bed is used for preventing bedsores, back, butt, and upper body discomfort. The bed could be any size in length and width to suit any place that has a patient or patients. The invention includes a dialysis machine and its system components. The invention reduces injury, improves arterial flow with a needle adjustable reducer, and prevents patients from falling with a side bed. Further, the bedding system rotates and thereby prevents injuries such as back and shoulder pain.

Referring now to Figures 1 through 22, the invention may include the following components:

10 – the headboard

12 – the footboard

14 – the sliding platform

16 – the handles

18 – the stationary platform

20 – the base

22 – the wheels

24 – the side panel

26 – the side panel base platform

28 – the hinge pin

30 – the hinge pin blocks

32 – the hinges

34 – the needle adjuster

36 – piece A

38 – piece B

40 – the butterfly clamp

42 – the needle

44 – tube A

46 – tube B

48 – the armrest

50 – the pants and shirt

52 – the zippers

54 – the cleaning system

56 – the prescription tray

58 – the prescription caps

60 – the dialysis machine

62 – the prescription supports (please note A)

64 – the prescription tray B

66 – the patient

68 – the ware and mirror

The answer and solution you seek elm>pn

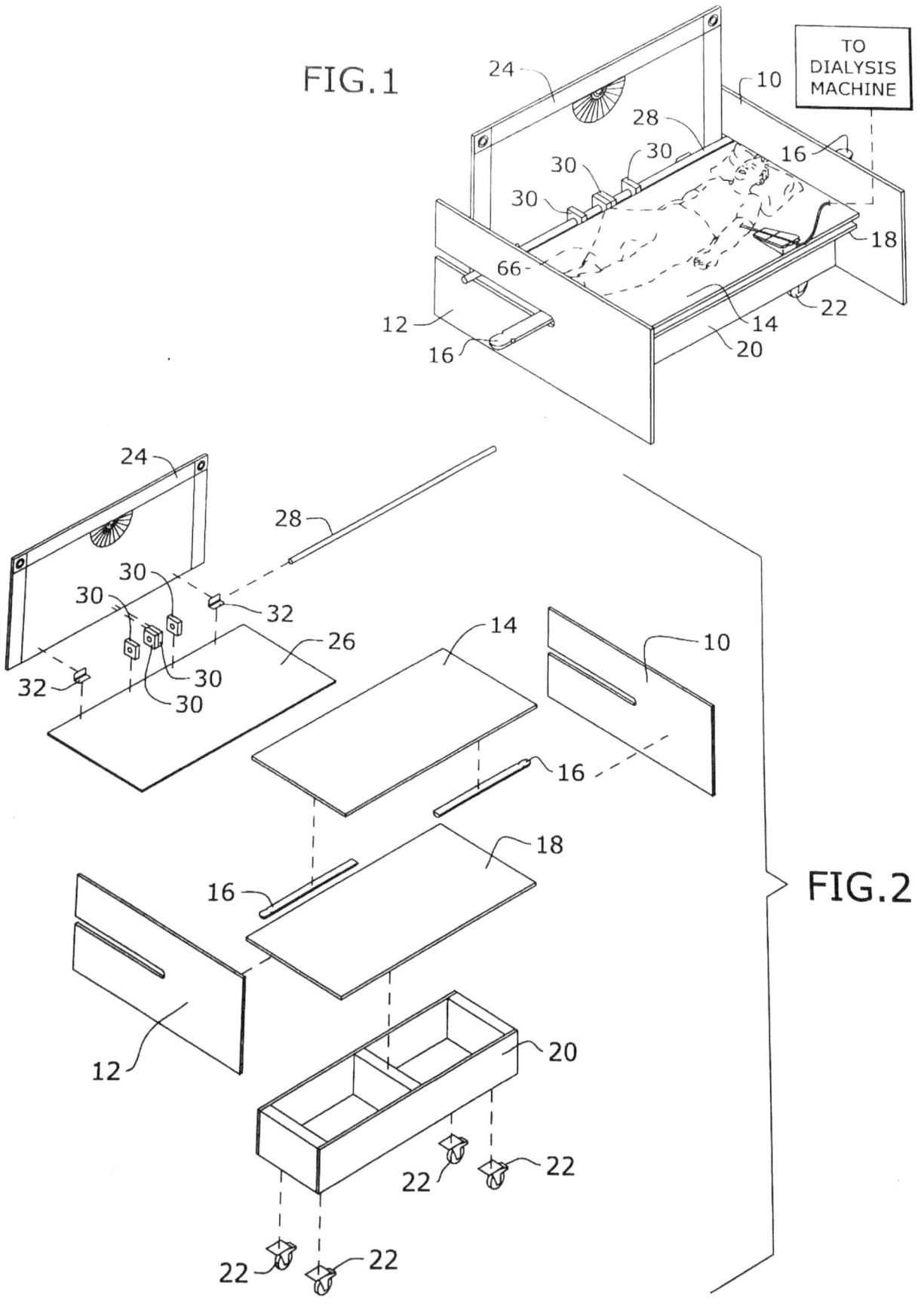

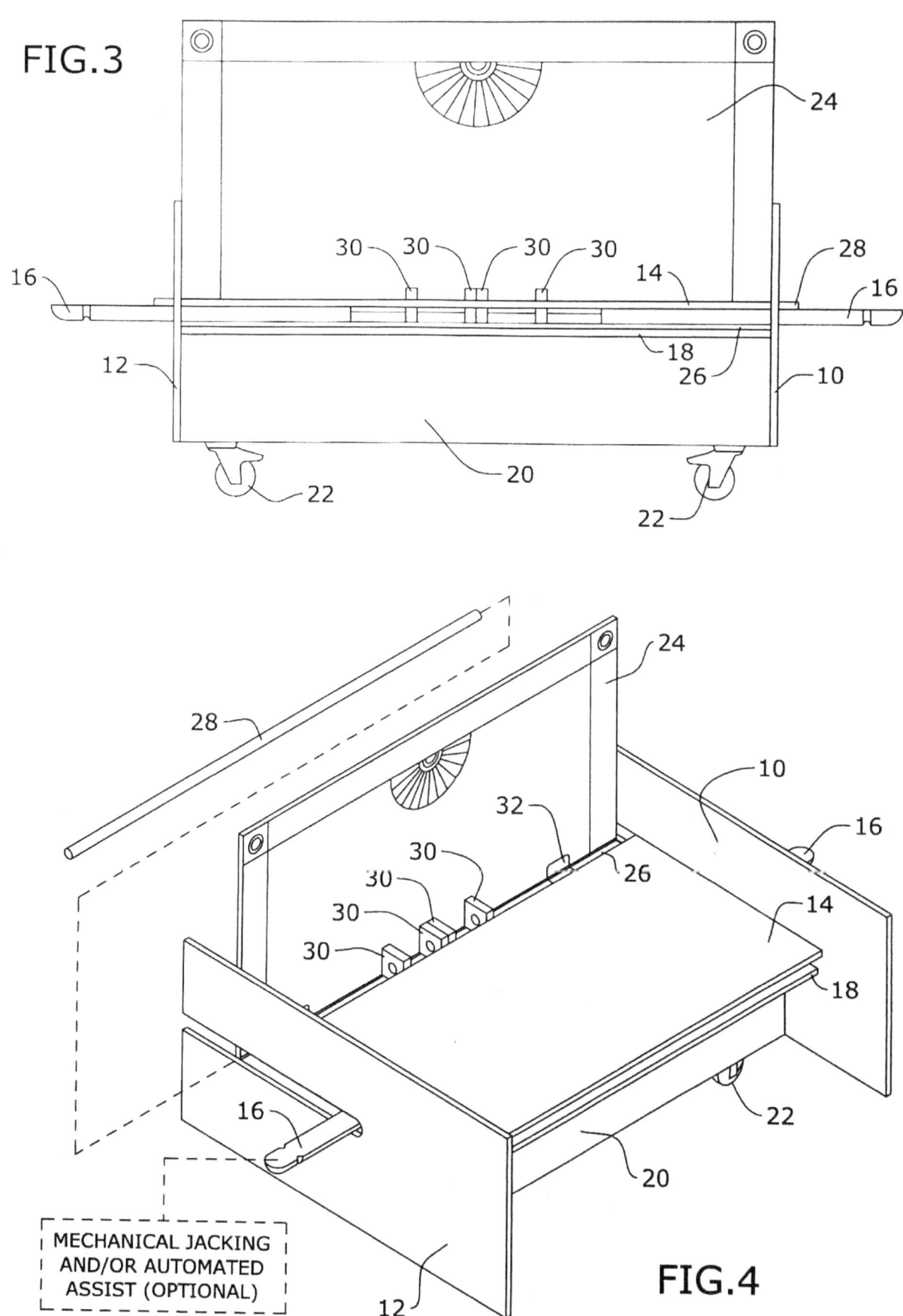

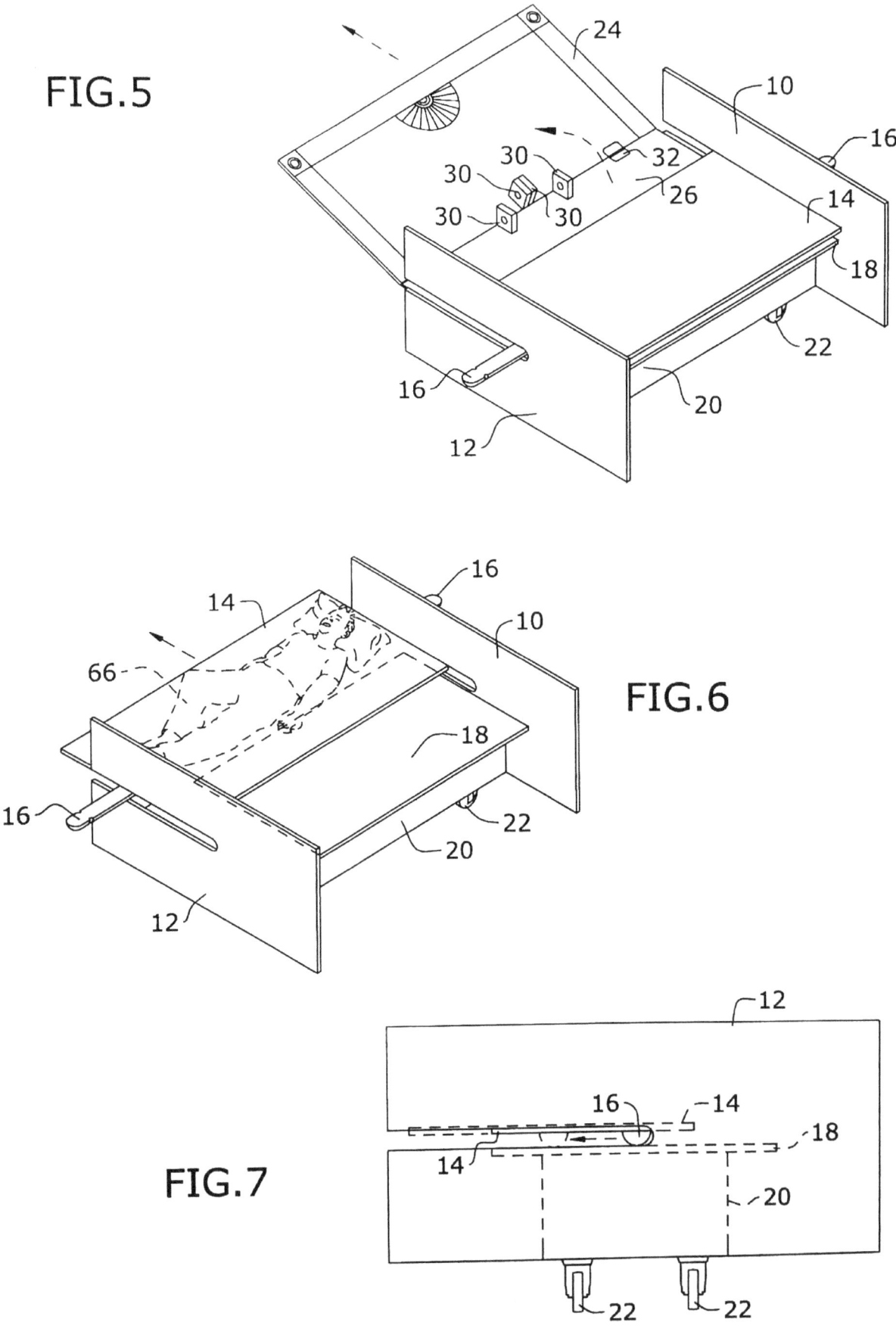

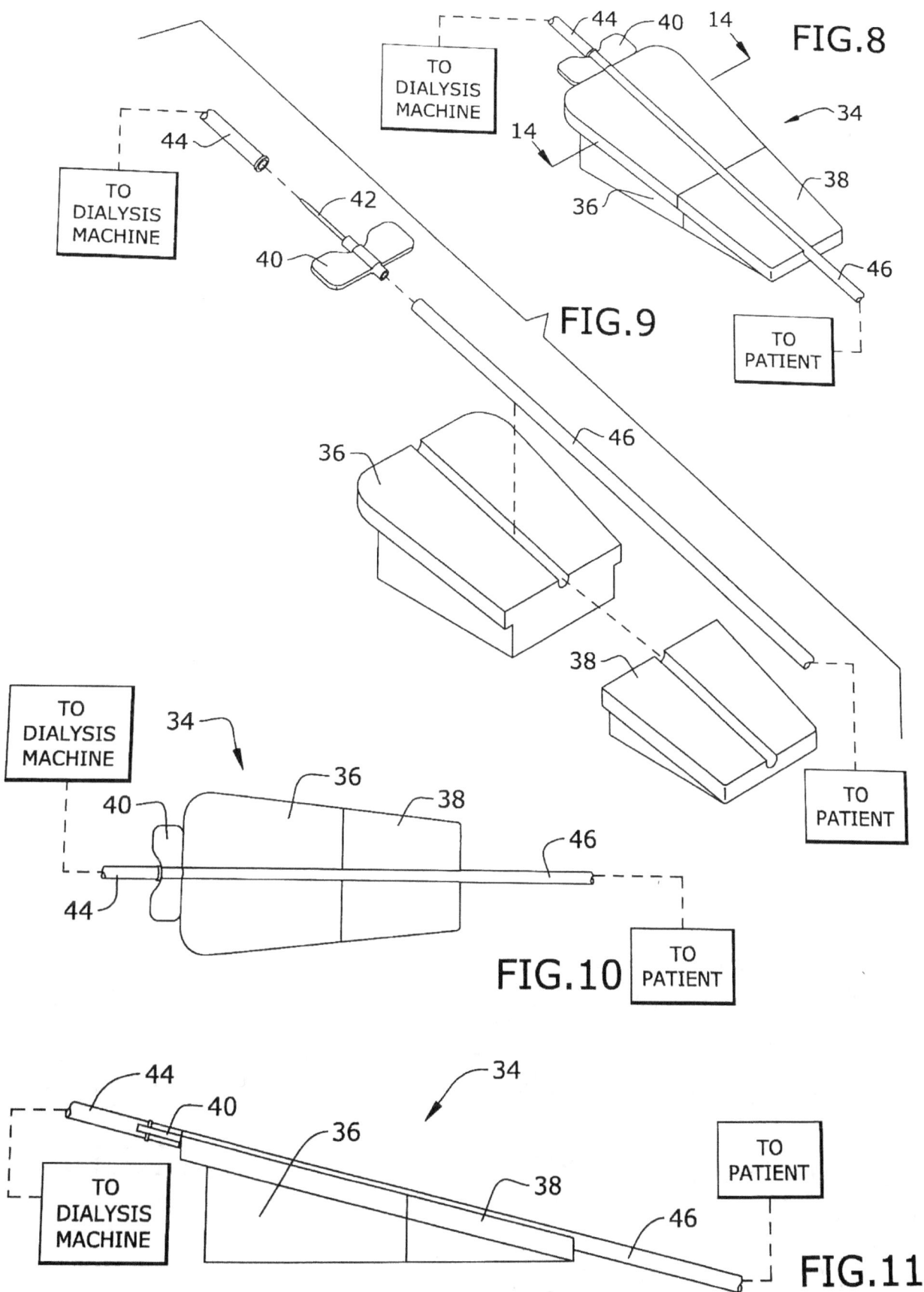

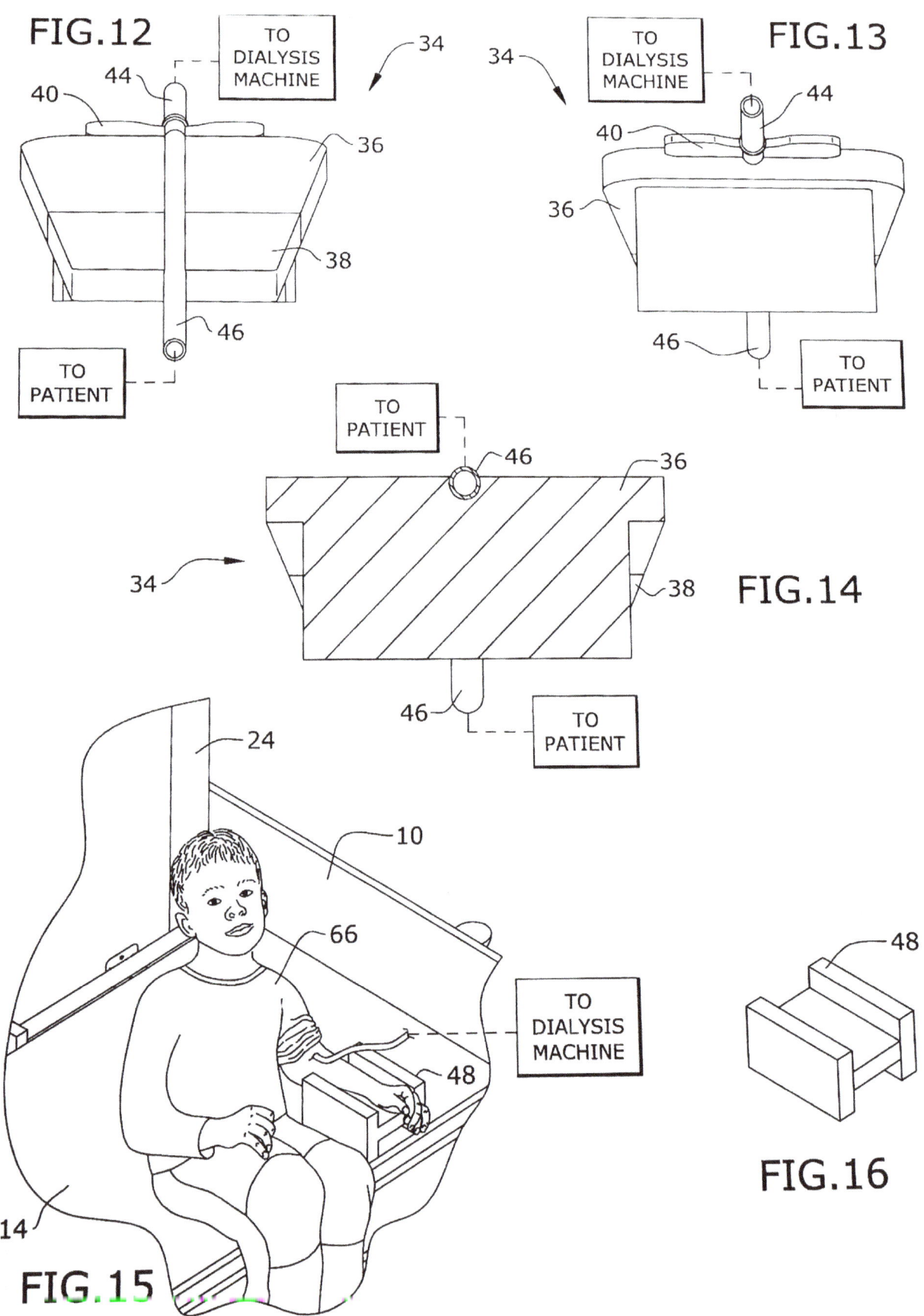

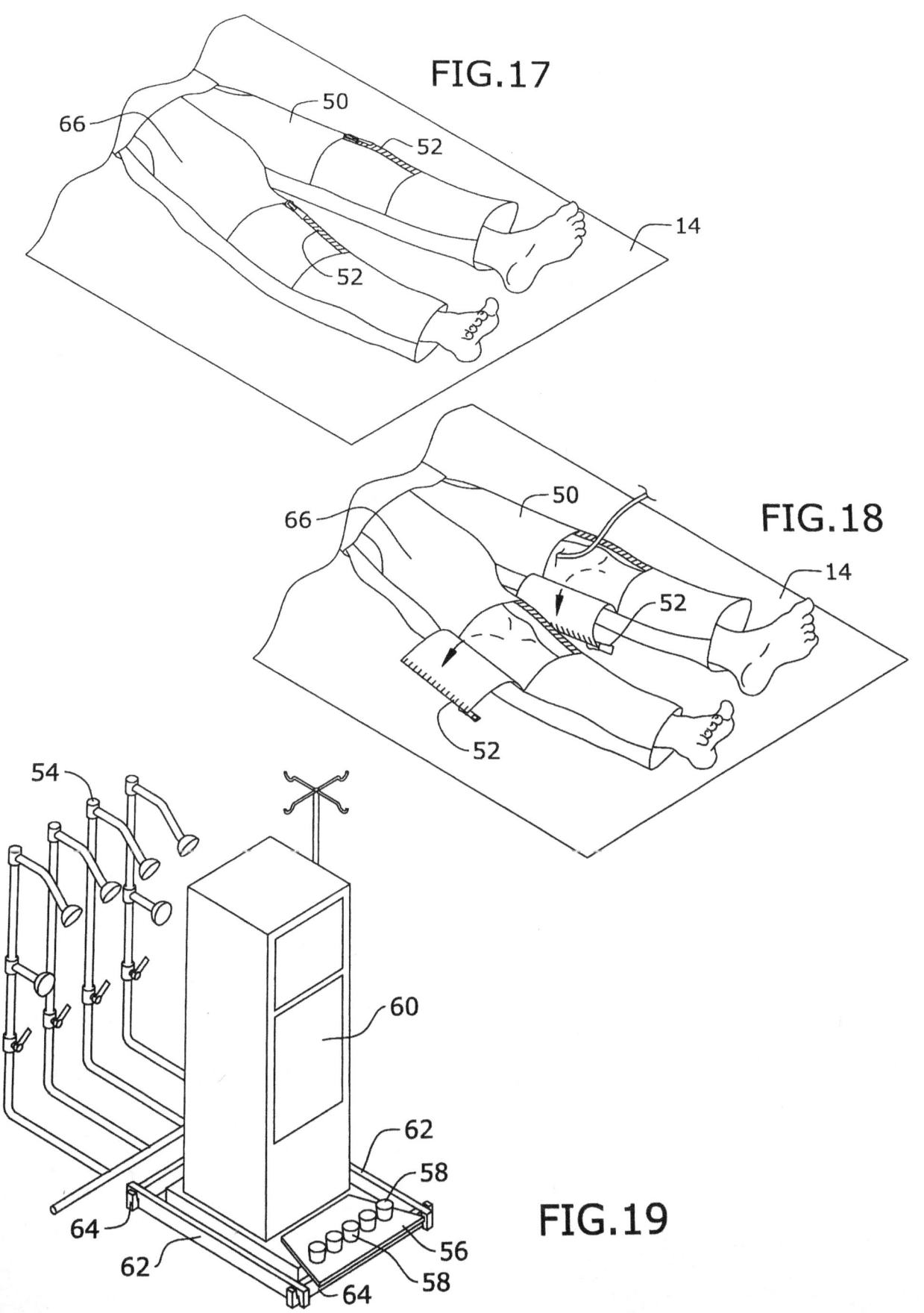

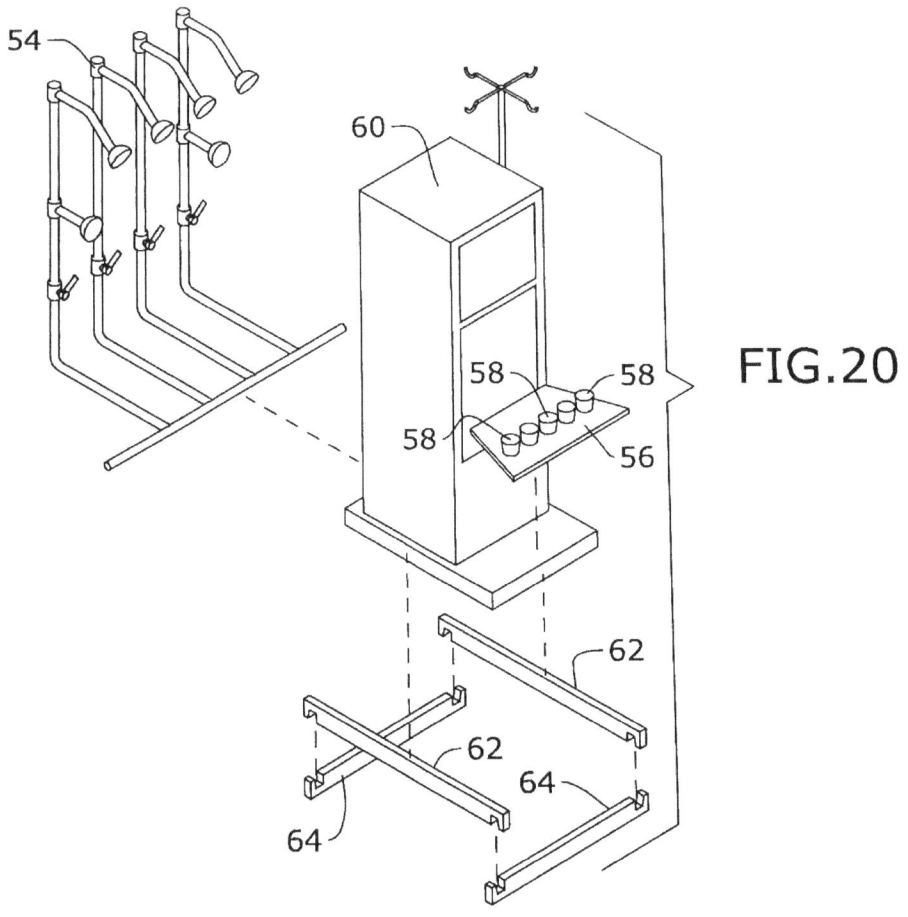

FIG.20

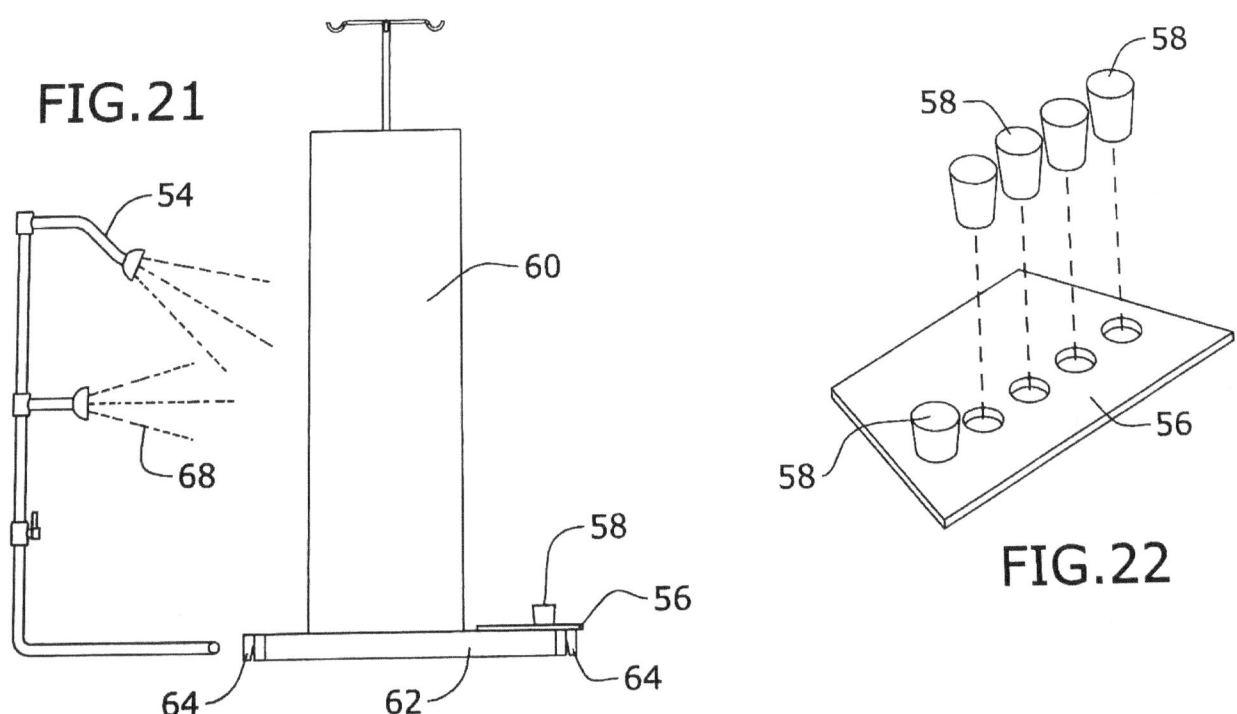

FIG.21

FIG.22

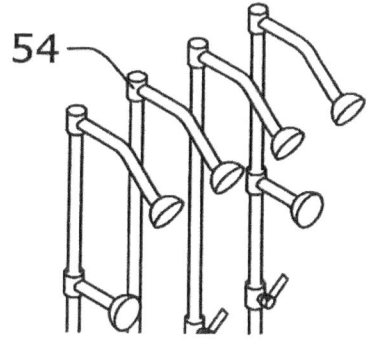
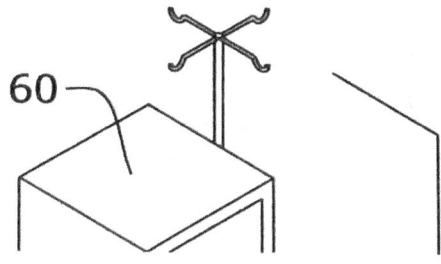

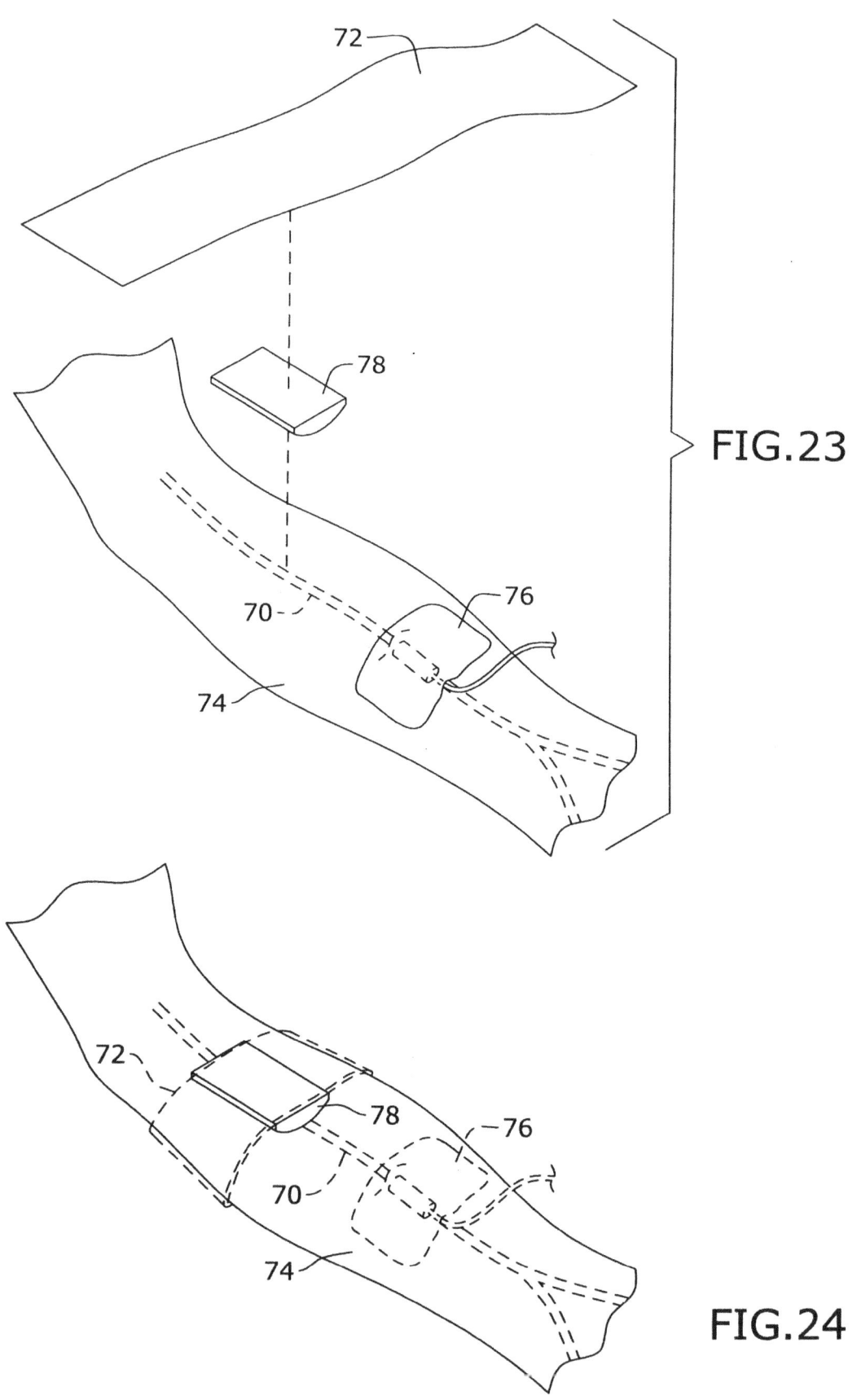

FIG.23

FIG.24

The lower part of the bed is called the semi-rotation circle connecting the headboard. The purpose is to allow the core bed to rotate side by side, allowing circulation to the body and heart, and minimizing cramping. This is how to reduce sores on the right side or left side of the body. The core bed and its head part is the main rotating part. The sliding part, which is also the core bed, with the assistance of trained medical staff (including paramedics, technicians, and nurses) allows the core bed to move up and slide to the right or left. This is how to move the patient from the aid of the core bed to an ordinary bed, which will prevent medical staff from injuring their back. With the aid of a power or manual jack, the core bed lifts up. Medical staff manually slides the bed to an ordinary bed. The medical set includes the following components:

Headboard size, 4 feet wide (this may be larger), 6 feet long, height 42 inches. The dimensions differ based on customer demand. The space to the right or left side of the lower part of the headboard with the semicircle can be 2 inches. The semicircle can be any circumference—the size of a penny, dime, nickel, quarter, and the like. The core bed may include a motor connecting to the core bed headboard that rotates the bed side to side. The jack piece, which is under the bed, is used to lift up the bed automatically or manually. The main dialysis bed can be made with wood, plastic, aluminum, copper, iron, or the like and allows a patient to enjoy an effective treatment. This bed would reduce cramping of the legs and abdomen and reduce side, neck, and shoulder discomfort. To manufacture the bed, various tools and equipment may be used, such as screws, screwdrivers, hand or electrical saw, hammer, wrenches, band saw, etc. To make the semicircle for the headboard lower part, a cut of the size of a ball of a quarter is made whereas the core headboard would be one inch, round in shape, allowing the core bed to rotate when connecting to the rotation motor. Connecting an electrical jack or manual under the core headboard fits the semicircle, lubricating to allow smooth ratio of the automatic or manual system. A plywood sheet, plastic sheet, or metal plate can be used to manufacture this innovation.

Medical staff are trained by WUFO Technologies staff. The feet of the core bed has movable wheels to allow the bed to move from one side to another side of the room without having to take apart the core bed. The main dialysis machine may include a bottom to cover the base in order to prevent debris from getting under the front of the wheel of the dialysis machine. The hole in the top of the covering in front of the machine is to place medications or a pot of flowers for decorative purposes. The top base could have other useful purposes. The front covering base is to prevent debris from getting under the wheel. The mirror on top of the machine allows a back view of other patients behind you. These parts can be made with a metal plate, plastic, wood, copper, or the like. An L-shaped holder may be connected to the back mirror in place, and the mirror could be any size and length. The material used to mount the mirror may include wood, plastic, metal, copper, aluminum, and the like.

The invention may include components for shoulder comfort. This part is to provide a more comfortable hand position allowing hand, neck, and shoulder flexibility. The length may be 12 inches or longer and 5 1/2 inches wide. Materials may include plastic, wood, metal, ceramic clay, and the like. These parts can be mounted with screws or glue if desired. The sizes mentioned can be adjusted. The upper circle holder may be a piece at the top and bottom and contain holes for screws to keep the safe side secure, total screws two: one screw up and one screw down. The bar safe could be more based on manufacturing choices and cost. The upper circle holder is mounted 4 inches from the bottom lower corner of the safe side. The lower circle holder may be placed at the corner of the safe side and may include two or more.

The needle adjuster is used for safety. The purpose of the part is to prevent the needles from dislodging from the insertion site. The part is 1 inch long, 1 inch wide, and 1 inch thick, with a center groove which may be 5 centimeters in depth and 5 centimeters in width. The needle's line is put inside the center hole for adjusting the needle's position and reducing the likelihood of the needle coming out of the insertion site. This allows greater blood flow or medication. This part can be increased or decreased in size. It can be made with wood, ceramic clay, metal, copper, aluminum, plastic, fabric, and the like. The invention may include a shower. The purpose of this part is to carry in these long standing pipes that are up vertically and lie on the floor or the ground 4 to 3 inches. These pipes could be 1 inch to 100 feet tall. One main pipe would be connected to the public or commercial water sewer via an automatic pump or not automatic to draw water into the main pipe. At this point water will be distributed to the main four pipes that stand vertically and lie horizontally for clean water.

This vertical and horizontal pipe could be aluminum, plastic, iron, copper, and the like. To build this part copper pipe is needed 5 feet tall and to 100 feet long. The needle adjuster can be used in the medical field. This bed can be used for specific purposes, which would help reduce bedsores because of its specific design. The global army can use the blood reducer to save a person from bleeding. The medical bed would improve productivity not just in medical settings but also in hospitals, nursing homes, or private homes. The invention reduces the amount of effort it takes to transfer a patient from one bed to another. This system is the safest and fastest. It should be understood, of course, that the foregoing relates to exemplary embodiments of the invention and that modifications may be made without departing from the spirit and scope of the invention.

THE SYSTEM ELEMENTS:

PATENT A
511893709

Medical Bed—brief description of the drawings

Fig. 1 is a perspective view of the invention in use.

Fig. 2 is a close-up view of the invention.

Fig. 3 is a front view of the invention.

Fig. 4 is a perspective view of the invention illustrating the hinge pin being removed.

Fig. 5 is a perspective view of the bed illustrating the side panel and side panel base platform being removed.

Fig. 6 is a perspective view of the invention shown in use illustrating the active platform being moved; side panel and side panel base platform removed for clarity.

Fig. 7 is a mirror located on top of the dialysis machine.

is a side view of the invention illustrating the active platform being moved; side panel and side panel base platform removed for clarity.

Fig. 8 is a perspective view of the needle adjuster.

Fig. 9 is a close-up view of the needle adjuster.

Fig. 10 is a top view of the needle adjuster.

Fig. 11 is a side view of the needle adjuster.

Fig. 12 is a front view of the needle adjuster.

Fig. 13 is a rear view of the needle adjuster.

Fig. 14 is a section view of the needle adjuster taken 14-14 in Fig. 8.

Fig. 15 is a perspective view of the armrest shown in use.

Fig. 16 is a perspective view of the armrest.

Fig. 17 is a perspective view of the pants illustrating the zipper closed.

Fig. 18 is a perspective view of the pants illustrating the zipper opened, shown in use and shirt in use.

Fig. 19 is a perspective view of the cleaning system, the perspective tray, and the tray supports shown in use.

Fig. 20 is a close-up view of the cleaning system, the prescription tray, and the tray supports.

Fig. 21 is a side view of the cleaning system, the prescription tray, and the tray supports shown in use.

Fig. 22 is a close-up view of the prescription tray.

DETAILED DESCRIPTION OF THE INVENTION The following detailed description is of the best currently contemplated modes of carrying out exemplary embodiments of the invention. The description is not to be taken in a limiting sense, but is made merely for the purpose of illustrating the general principles of the invention. The invention includes a sliding bed for medical use for all patients.

The bed is used for preventing bed sore, back butt and upper body discomforts. The bed could be any size in length and width(wide)to suit any place that has a patient or patients. The present invention includes a dialysis machine and its system components. The problem the Present invention solves is it reduces repetitive injury ,injury improves arterial flow, with a needle adjuster, BLD reducer, prevents patients from falling with a side bed. Further, the bedding system rotates and thereby prevents injuries such as back and shoulder pain.

Referring now to Figures 1 through 22. The invention may include the following components: 10 – the headboard; 12 – the footboard; 14 – the sliding platform; 16 – the handles; 18 – the stationary platform; 20 – the base; 22 – the wheels; 24 – the side panel; 26 – the side panel base platform; 28 – the hinge pin; 30 – the hinge pin blocks; 32 – the hinges; 34 – the needle adjuster; 36 – piece A; 38 – piece B; 40 – piece of the butterfly clamp; 42 – the needle; 44 – tube A; 46 – tube B; 48 – the armrest; 50 – the pants and shirt; 52 – the zippers; 54 – the cleaning system; 56 – the prescription tray; 58 – the prescription caps; 60 – the dialysis machine; 62 – the prescription supports (please note A); 64 – the prescription tray B; 66 – the patient; 68 – the ware

The lower part of the bed is called the semi rotation circle connecting head bed. The purpose is to allow the core bed to rotate side by side. This rotation is what will allow the bed to move side to side allowing circulation to the body and heart minimizing cramping. This is how to reduce soars on the right side or left side of the human body. The Core bed and its head part is the main rotating part. The sliding part which is also the core bed with assistance of train of train medical staff which include Paramedics, Technician, Nurses allowing the core bed to move up an slide to the right or left. This how to move the patient from the aid of the core bed to an ordinary bed, which will prevent medical staff from injuring their back. With the aid of a power or manual jack the core bed lift up. Medical staff manually slides the bed to an ordinary bed. The medical set includes the following components Head bed size, 4 feet wide, this may be lager, length 6 feet long height 42 inches. The dimension different base on customer Demand. The space to the right or left side of the lower part of head bed with semi-circle could be is 2 inches. The semi-circle could be any circumference.

Such as the size of a penny, dime, nickel, quarter and like. The core bed may include a motor connecting to the core bed head, and rotates the bed to the side. The jack piece which is under the bed is used to lift up the bed automatically or manually. The main dialysis bed which could be made with woods, plastic, aluminum, copper, iron, or the like allows a patient to be able to enjoy an effect treatment. This bed would reduce cramping of the leg and abdominal, side discomfort, neck and shoulder discomfort. To manufacture the bed various tools and equipment may be used, such as screws, screwdrivers, hand saw or electrical, hammer, wrenches, band saw and the like. To make the semi-circle for the head bed lower part a cut of the size of a ball of a quarter is made whereas the core head bed would be size one inch round in shape allowing the core bed to rotate when connecting to the rotation Motor. Connecting an electrical jack or manual under the core bed head fits the semi-circle lubricating to allow smooth ratio of the automatic or manual system. A plywood sheet, plastic, sheet, or metal plate can be used to manufacture this innovation. Medical Staffs is trained by WUFO Technologies staff. The feet of the core bed has movable wheels to allow the bed to move from one side to another side of room to another side without having to take apart the core bed. The main Dialysis Machine may include a bottom to cover the base in order to prevent debris from getting under the front of the wheel of the dialysis machine. The hole in the top of the covering front of the machine is to place gallons of medications which are used in medical treatment or pot of flower for decorative purposes. The top base could have other useful purposes and the rest of its usefulness. Front covering base is to prevent debris from getting under the wheel. The mirror on top of the machine allows back view of other patients behind you. These parts can be made not just metal plate, plastic or wood, copper and the like. A L shaped holder may be connect to the back mirror in place, and the size of the mirror could be any size and length.

Mount the mirror may include wood plastic, metal, copper aluminum and the like. The present invention may include components for shoulder comfort. This part is to provide a more comfortable hand position allowing hand, neck and shoulder flexibility. The length may be 12 inches or longer and 5 1/2 inches wide. Materials may include plastic, wood metal, ceramic clay and the like. These parts can be mounted with screws or glue if desire. The sizes mentioned can be adjusted. The upper circle holder may be a piece at the top and bottom and contains holes for screws to keep the safe side secure, total screws two one screw up and one screw down. The bar safe could be more based on manufacturing choices and cost. The upper circle holder is mounted 4 inches from the bottom lower corner of safe side. The lower circle holder may be placed at the corner of safe side and may include two or more. The needle adjuster is used for safety. The purpose of the part is to prevent the needles from dislodge(coming out from insertion site).The part is 1 inch length,1 inch wide and 1 inch in thick, with a center grove which may be 5 centimeter in depth and 5 centimeter in width. The needles lines is put inside the center hole for adjusting the needles position and reducing the likelihood of the needles from coming out of the insertion site. Which allows greater blood flow or medication. This part can increase in size or decrease in size. This part can be made with wood, ceramic clay, metal, copper, aluminum, plastic fabric and the like. The present invention may include a shower. The purpose of this part is carry in these Long standing pipe that are up vertically and lay on the floor or the ground 4 to 3 inches and these pipe could be 1 inch to 100 feet tall. One main pipe would be connected to the public or commercial water sewer via an automatic pump or not automatic to draw water into the main pipe, at this point water will be distributed to the main four pipe that are stand vertically and lay horizontally the aim for these system is to water clean. This vertical and horizontal pipe could be aluminum, plastic, iron copper and the like. To build this part copper pipe is needed five feet tall and to feet long. The needle adjuster can be use in the medical field, this bed can be used for specific purpose, which would ad in reducing bed sore because of it specific design. The Global army can use the blood reducer to save a person from bleeding. The medical bed would improve productivity not just in medical setting also in hospital, a private nursing homes or private homes. The present invention reduces the amount of effort it takes to transfer a patient from on bed to another this system is the safest and fastest. It should be understood, of course, that the foregoing relates to exemplary embodiments, of the invention and that modifications may be made without departing from the spirit and scope of the invention.

www.ingramcontent.com/pod-product-compliance
Lightning Source LLC
Chambersburg PA
CBHW062209220526
45470CB00009B/2984